Choose Your Personal Diet

Gunter Schaule BSc MBA
Consultant:
Professor U de Brentani PhD

ISBN 9781512218992

Contents

1. THE SCIENTIFIC CONCEPT

Science has now determined what makes us fat. It is not the fat in food, but sugar and starch. It is not calories that count, but another nutritional measure, the Glycemic Index (GI). The GI counts the sugar level in our blood.

That has made it simpler. To stay slim, we don't have to starve ourselves with low calorie regimes. We only have to select the right food and we can eat plenty of it.

We all have different body-energy requirements, depending on our lifestyle. People who work physically, and sporty individuals need sustained energy. The Glycemic Index identifies the food that provides sustained power.
What we all want to avoid are short energy spikes followed by fatigue and hunger pangs.

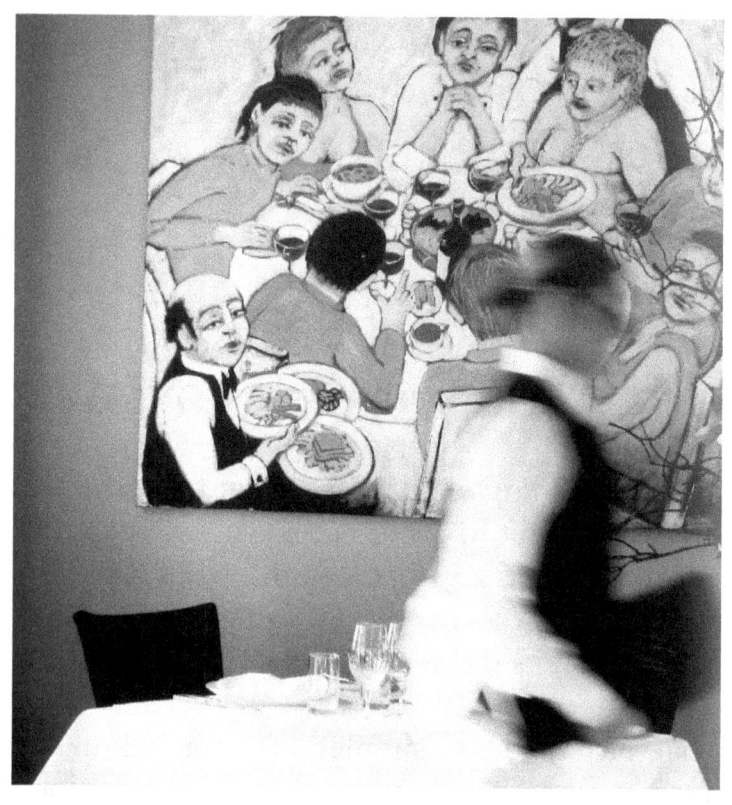

Many myths abounded in the past about weight control. People moved from one esoteric diet fad to another, often without success.

Here are these simple scientific facts.

1) If your food and drink produce more energy than you need within a limited timeframe, the excess energy gets converted into fat and stored as body fat. That's how our body developed when we

were cave-dwellers, to produce reserves for famines.

2) The extra energy gets only produced by sugar in our food and drinks, and by starch in the food. Starch gets converted into blood sugar (Glucose).

3) Protein in our food produces no energy. It builds muscles, but if not required, it gets eliminated.

So all excess energy comes from sugar and starch. When they get converted and deposited as fat, they also help storing away the fat in our food.

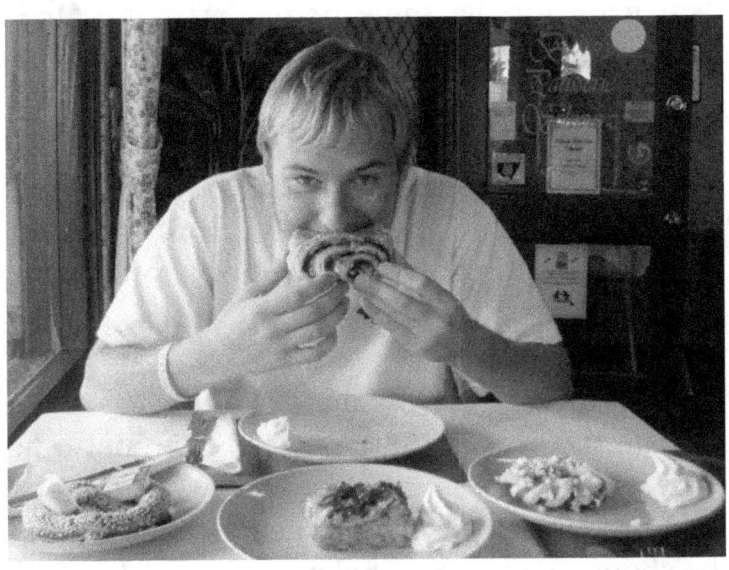

2. LIFESTYLE AND ENERGY NEED

You probably won't worry too much about your weight, if you jog for an hour a day, or you walk for the same period or more. Or if you work on a construction site and you are in motion all day long. You need all the energy you can get and you can eat anything you like without gaining weight. Even then, it will be good for you to know what type of food gives you sustained energy. This will be shown in the tables below.

On the other hand, if you are sitting most of the day, in the office, in the car, and in front of the TV, you burn less energy, and you need food that produces less power. The best choices will be shown in the tables below.

This is where many of us work nowadays:

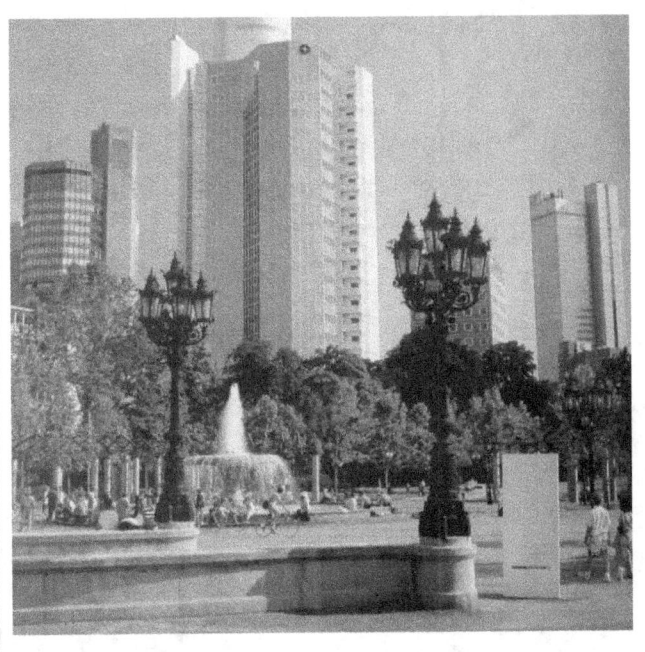

We need to know how much energy is produced by the specific food and drink we consume. The food that produces lots of power we have to avoid if we don't excrete ourselves. The good news is, food that produces little energy we can eat in abundance! We have a wide and attractive selection.

How do we know the difference in food energy? It is not measured in Calories. Science has defined a new measure for the food energy in our bloodstream, the Glycemic Index (GI).

To briefly demonstrate the difference between Calories and the Glycemic Index, for example, a **steak** has lots of Calories, but its proteins produce no blood sugar to give us energy, so its **GI is zero**.

It is up to us to choose the food and drink that matches our energy requirement. The food tables following later provide all the GI details.

This is how people used to live. It required lots of work energy. Our body developed for that, and for fat storage to survive famines.

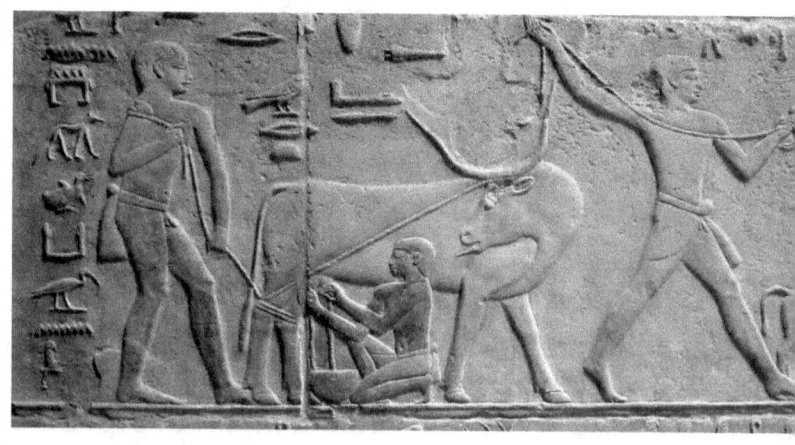

We probably know whether on average we are burning lots of power or not so much. In addition, the examples below can give us an idea of some typical energy requirements in the old measure of calories. A person of average weight typically uses up only a moderate amount of energy. The second table puts it in perspective to the calorie production of some food.

Going for a half hour walk burns just 75 calories (cal).

Cycling in a flat area for half an hour uses up 110 cal.

Light swimming in temperate water, ½ an hour, 150 cal.

Moderate conditioning exercise, half an hour, 200 cal.

Jogging for half an hour burns 330 cal.

In comparison, eating gives us energy as follows:

One thick slice of white bread produces 100 cal.

A simple bowl of cornflakes is 130 cal.

Just one bagel gives us energy of 140 cal.

A serving of boiled pasta has a power input of 330 cal.

A serving of roasted potatoes loads us up with 420 cal.

See the related GI values and their ranking in the tables further below.

3. HOW GAING WEIGHT WORKS

It's not really how much we eat, but exactly what we eat. Technically, the process runs as follows. Some types of carbohydrates raise our blood sugar level, calling the hormone INSULIN into the blood stream. Insulin deposits the blood sugar (Glucagon) into our muscle cells for any required energy production, and it converts the excess blood sugar into fat for storage purposes. Insulin also deposits the *fat* that is in our food into fat pockets. Therefore, without a raised blood sugar level and without increased Insulin, fat cannot be retained; it gets eliminated. Fat is only fattening if consumed with carbs that raise our blood sugar level.

The FIRST SECRET is: Not all excess calories (e.g., proteins) get stored as fat.

The SECOND SECRET is: Only certain carbohydrates call enough Insulin into the blood stream to create fat pockets.

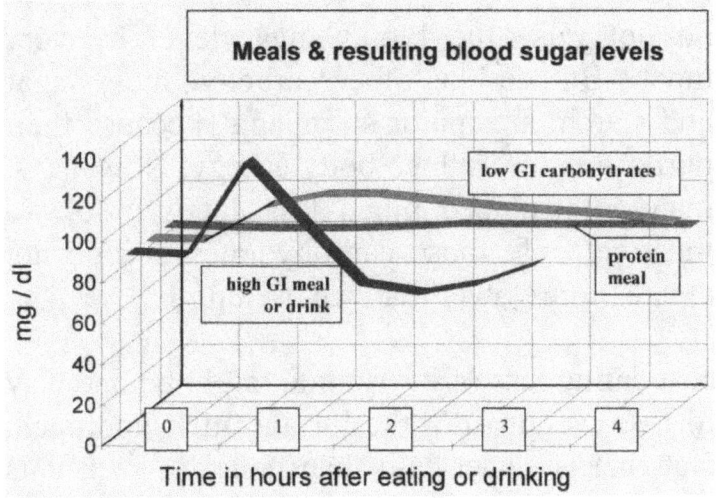

Meals & resulting blood sugar levels

low GI carbohydrates

high GI meal or drink

protein meal

mg / dl

Time in hours after eating or drinking

It's important to realize that not all foods make us fat. As noted above, only certain types of carbohydrates call enough Insulin into the blood stream to create fat pockets. So, the key question is: What kind of carbohydrates are these?

ONLY FOOD THAT RAISES OUR BLOOD SUGAR TO HIGH LEVELS QUICKLY can make us fat!

Scientists have identified a that measure — the GLYCEMIC INDEX (GI) — which tells us to what extent the blood sugar level is raised by various types of foodstuffs or meals. This is illustrated in the diagram above.

Protein foods do <u>not</u> raise our blood sugar level at all (see diagram). Also, *some* carbohydrates do <u>not</u> raise the blood sugar level by very much. But certain other carbohydrates, sugar and starch, are major stimulants, because their purpose is to produce body energy. Nowadays, many of us need much less energy! So, we must eat only those carbohydrates that do not create more power than we use up.

Just eating less of everything might be one way to lose weight. It's the hit and miss approach. But that is easier said than done! In fact, it is quite unrealistic! This is because it leads to a 'yo-yo' effect:

Our body is used to its customary intake of calories. If we switch to eating less, our body senses hard times. Because it runs on auto-pilot to ensure its survival when things get tough, the body puts on more reserves, giving us less energy for daily activities. Weak and depressed, we are in despair and end up eating more in order to feel better again. This is the yo-yo effect of a reduced calorie diet.

So, counting calories helps very few people to lose weight in the long term!

Besides the yo-yo effect, most of us can't fight off the temptation presented by all the glorious food and drink around us. We don't want to miss out on the joy of eating! We don't want to give up the social pleasure of sharing a nice meal with family and friends. In fact, good eating is part of a civilised society.

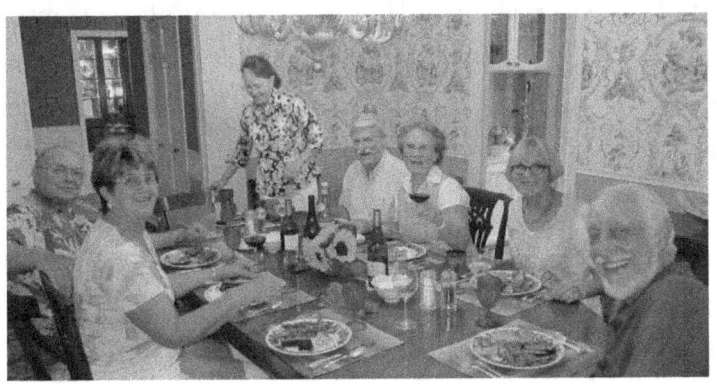

4. CARBS AIN'T CARBS!

Only 'certain' carbohydrates raise our blood sugar level, while others have almost no effect. And that is the key to maintaining or losing weight.

There is a huge difference between types of carbo-hydrates. Some get absorbed quickly by our body, creating a blood sugar spike that cannot be easily reduced through energy use. Others create almost
no blood sugar, while still others get digested slowly, releasing energy over a long period of time.

The Glycemic Index (GI) tells us by how much the blood sugar level increases in the first hours after eating. The GI ranges between 0 and about 100. A low GI means a low increase in blood sugar level (Glucose), and this means that less excess energy and fat will be stored as fat reserves. Only too much high-GI food and drink makes us fat.

So, we don't have to starve ourselves! WE CAN EAT PLENTY OF <u>LOW-GI</u> FOOD and feel satisfied all day.

Check it out in the four tables that follow, which go from a GI value of 0 to 100, and in extreme cases even above.

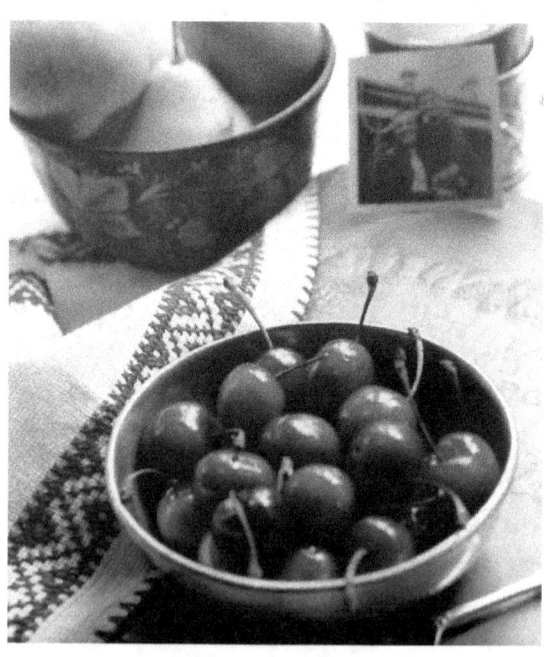

TABLE 1

EAT TO LOSE WEIGHT

GI	
0	Water
0	Dry Wine
0	All Proteins, like: Meat, Fish, Cheese
0	Green Beans
0	Spinach, Rocket
0	Lettuce, Celery
0	Cucumber
6	Avocado
10	Mushrooms
10	Peppers, Onions
10	Broccoli
14	Natural Yoghurt
14	Peanuts
15	Tomatoes

GI value	
16	Raw Carrots
22	Cashew Nuts
22	Cherries
24	Milk, low fat
24	Plums
25	Grapefruit
27	Kidney Beans
30	Lentils
30	Dried Apricots
30	All Bran Cereal
33	Yoghurt
36	Chickpeas
38	Tomato Juice
38	Prem. Ice Cream
38	Apples, Pears
39	Strawberries
40	Milk, Soy Milk
40	Apple Juice

TABEL 2

Eat to maintain your weight and produce Sports Energy

GI (Glycemic Index)

41 Pumpernickel Bread
42 Peaches
43 Custard pudding
43 Ice cream
46 Macaroni
46 Grapes
46 Pizza
50 Whole rye bread
51 Mango
52 Kiwi Fruit
52 Oranges
52 Sushi Roll
52 Banana
53 Sweet potato
54 Sweet corn
55 Oatmeal Cookies
55 Oat bran cereal
56 Long grain rice
59 Danish muffin
59 Papaya
59 Pineapple
59 Brown rice

TABLE 3

EAT TO

PUT ON WEIGHT !

GI (Glycemic Index Value)

GI	Food	GI	Food
61	Hamburger Bun	67	Croissant
61	Ice Cream, regular	68	Taco Shells
63	Coca Cola	68	Cranberry Juice
64	Rye Bread	69	Special K Cereal
64	Shortbread	70	Weetabix
64	Raisins	71	Water Crackers
64	White Rice	72	Bagel
64	Beetroot	72	Pop Corn
65	Cantaloupe	73	Sultana Bran Cereal
65	Couscous	74	Sports Plus drink
66	Nutri Grain	75	French Fries
66	Instant Porridge	76	Waffles
66	Beer	76	Doughnut
		77	Choco Pops
		77	Vanilla Wafer

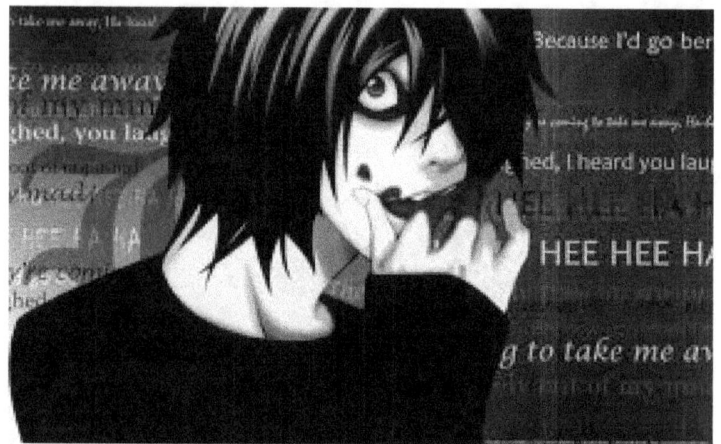

TABLE 4

SUPER

WEIGHT GAIN FOOD!

GI (Glycemic Index Value)		GI	
80	Wonderwhite Toast	90	Puffed Rice
80	Jelly Beans	91	Instant Rice
82	Rice Cakes	95	French Baguette
83	Cornflakes	102	Pancake Mix
85	Baked Potato	103	Dried Dates
85	Mashed Potatoes	109	Jasmine Rice
87	Corn Thins		

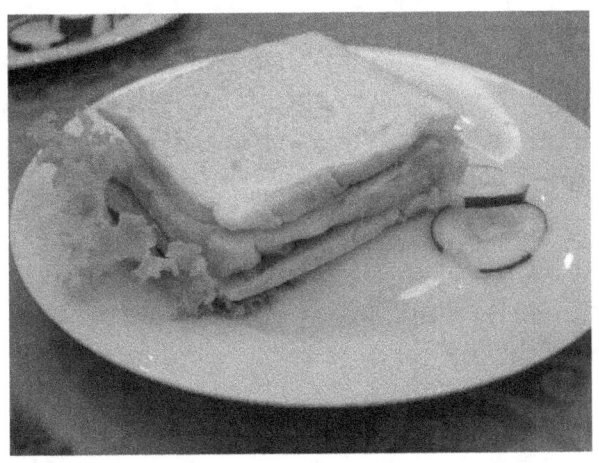

Seeing the everyday food in Table 4, it may be hard to believe that this is the main problem! We are so used to these items, but we have to rethink our eating habits drastically to fit a lifestyle of lower energy requirements. All we need for a healthy diet across all food categories we can find in Table 1. From these items we can practically eat as much as we like. The food in Table 2 we can eat occasionally. To lose weight, we must avoid everything in Tables 3 and 4. It's not hard, it's just a question of knowing it.

For sustained sports energy, avoid items in Table 4, which give you short term energy only. Tables 2 and 3 are the best for prolonged power output.

It is important to understand why there is such a wide range in GI values for carbohydrates. GI values depend on several things, including: sugar content, degree of food processing and refinement (e.g. highly milled flower, processed cornflakes, polished rice with the bran removed), and also on the molecular structure of the food (for example, potatoes get quickly digested by our body, and starch is converted to sugar and sent into the blood stream almost immediately, producing a lot of short-term energy).

You can see from the GI tables above that moderate climate fruits have relatively low GI values, while tropical fruits generally are high GI, due their greater sugar content and their less fibrous structure. Therefore, cut down on tropical fruits and eat plenty of moderate climate fruits and berries.

High GI food causes a lot of Insulin to be released into the blood. As shown in the diagram, this oversupply of Insulin works at lowering the glucose level to BELOW NORMAL. This creates HUNGER PANGS and starts a renewed cycle of over-eating, blood sugar excess, and too much Insulin production. In the medium term, this leads to overweight. In the longer run, it can dull the Insulin receptors on cells and lead to DIABETES 2, a debilitating disease that can cause kidney failure, heart problems, cancer and blindness.

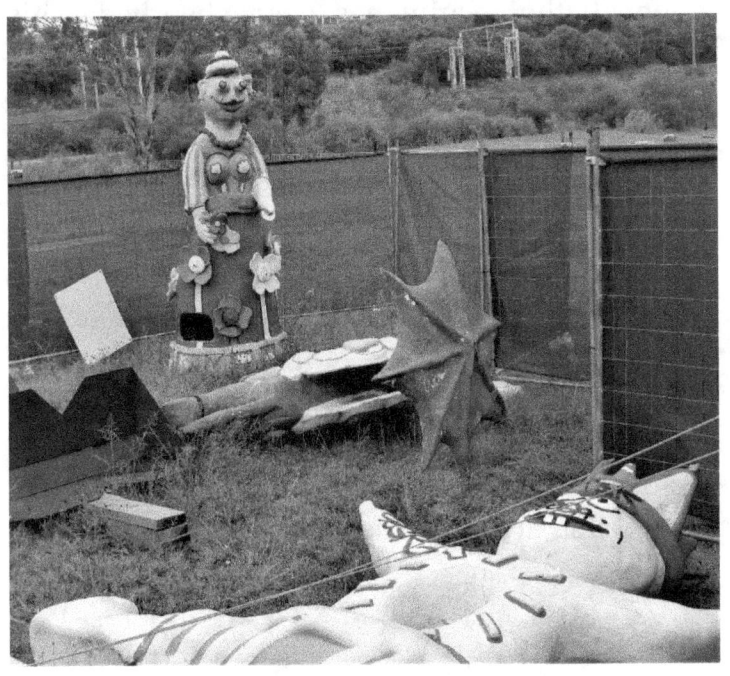

5. LOSING WEIGHT

As noted, Insulin *deposits* blood sugar into cells. Once the blood sugar is down to its normal level and there is no more Insulin in the blood stream, the body looks elsewhere for energy.

This is where another important hormone, called GLUCAGON, kicks in. Glucagon does exactly the opposite from Insulin; it **removes** fat from cells to produce energy. Therefore, shedding body fat doesn't start until a few hours after consuming carbohydrates — that is, when all the Insulin has been absorbed. This means that you need to take extended breaks between high insulin producing meals if you want to lose weight. In other words, no sweet or starchy snacks, or sweet drinks, etc. between meals.

But, because proteins produce no blood sugar and don't interfere with the fat burning action of Glucagon, you can enjoy other types of snacks such as cheese, eggs or meat cuts. As shown in the GI table above, various kinds of salads, or carrot and celery sticks have a very low GI and are ideal snacks.

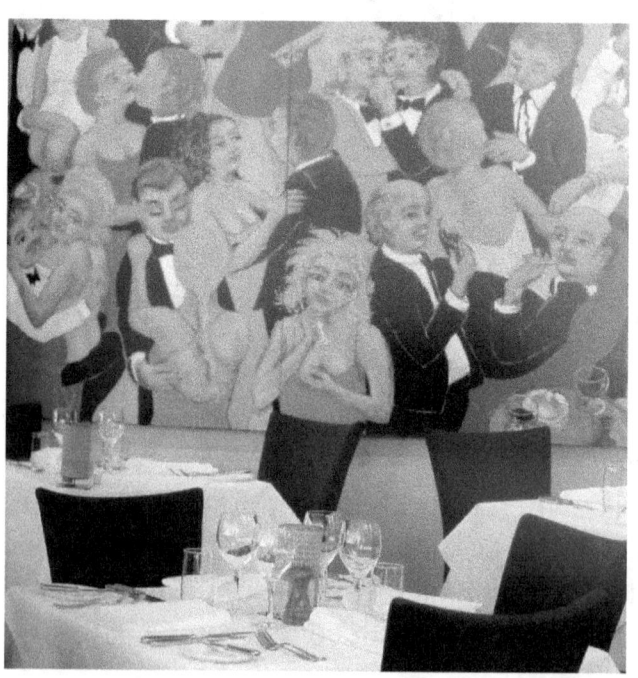

THE INSULIN – GLUCAGON INTERPLAY

Let's look at how Insulin and Glucagon play each other off in our daily lives. At all times, day or night, our body needs energy for its basic functioning at the BMR. During the day, our level of energy use varies, depending on what we are doing. The more physically active we are, the faster the Insulin level decreases, and the sooner the Glucagon hormone gets released. So, the higher the level of activity, the earlier fat burning starts. Even at night, this fat burning action continues. While we are asleep, about 3 hours after our last carbohydrate meal, Glucagon starts burning fat. To get fat burning started earlier in the evening, it is important to avoid those last cookies, chocolates, or sweet nightcaps.

If you had an opulent dinner, you may extend the Glucagon fat burning action, the 'fasting', by delaying break-fast or skipping breakfast all together, if you are awaking to a low energy morning at the PC or to sitting in the car. The old adage that breakfast is the most important meal applied to times when most people had physically demanding jobs. Nowadays, a good cappuccino can tie us over. The French tradition of just a coffee and a croissant looks like a good compromise.

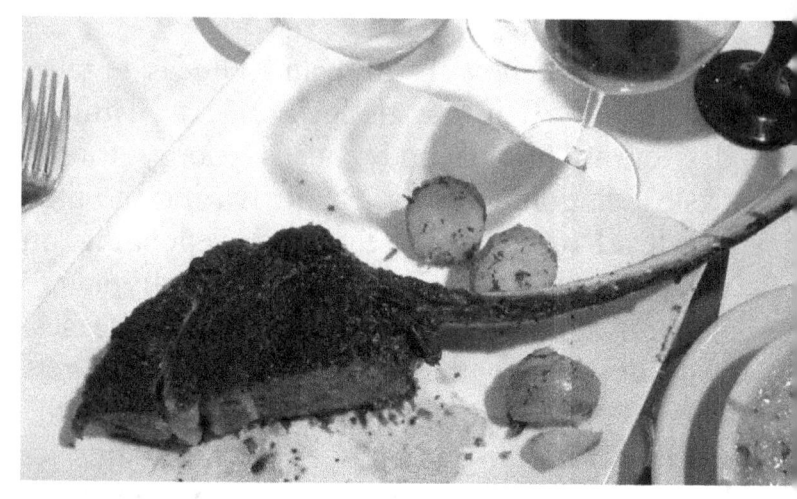

6.   D E T O X

Another factor impacting our bodily health, and weight, is the level of acidity in our system. We speak of the need for 'detoxification'. A primary reason for toxification of our body is slow digestion and delayed bowel evacuation. Some people are blessed with a fast and regular system. But if you are not, this is a cause for concern.

Slow digestion allows more food energy to be absorbed by the body, which leads to greater weight gain. The main reason for slow digestion is the highly processed nature of modern food. Finely milled flour, bread and breakfast cereals manufactured from highly processed and refined inputs, have had their fibres and natural coarseness removed. Similarly, white rice has its bran removed for appearance sake. As a result, the GI of many of our basic carbohydrates has been artificially increased to our detriment.

But even more devastating than causing slow digestion and therefore weight gain, the resulting waste product sits for too long in the last section of our intestines, the colon. There, it disseminates acidity and poisons our body.

Cancer of the colon is the leading cause of death in men.

We need to eat more fibrous and less refined food — as our ancestors did — to stimulate our digestion. And if that is not enough, laxatives may be required. There are excellent natural laxatives on the market.

Detoxification through regular bowel movements — at least once a day — should be an important goal if you want to avoid cancer and stop poisoning your body with acidity.

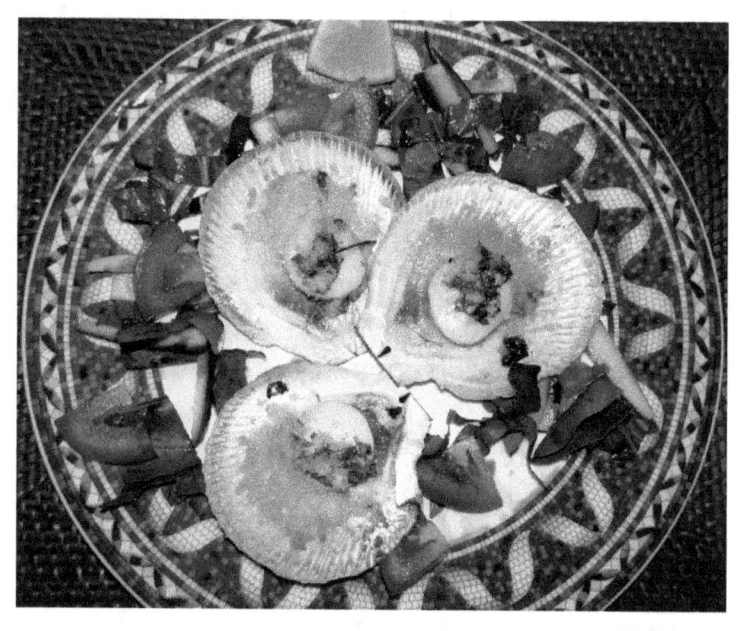

7.   E X E R C I S E

Exercise burns energy in our blood stream and it burns excess stored fat, which allows us to lose weight. Exercise also gives us a feeling of achievement, a positive outlook on life, and even fights depression. It increases our cardio-vascular activity, which is good for the longevity of our heart and our brain.

But, the fat burning effect of only casual exercise can be overestimated. The table in Section 2. above provides examples of the relative small power consumption of half hour exercises. If we want to keep or reduce your body weight, moderate exercise is only useful <u>without</u> additional eating or soft drinks. Only if you exercise intensely over longer periods of time you need extra energy through additional food intake. To use modest exercise as an excuse for additional eating is counter-productive.

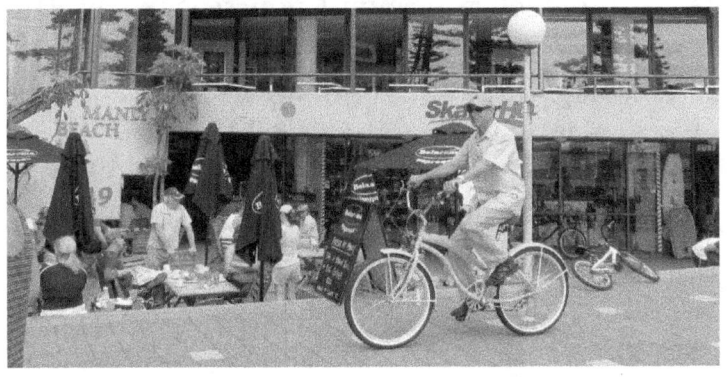

While many forms of exercise are good for our health, unless they are intensive, prolonged and regular, they are rarely enough to make us lose weight. In fact, it is much easier to reduce our energy intake by sticking to low GI food, than by trying to burn off the equivalent energy through exercise (as shown by the numeric examples in Section 2. above).

Also, some forms of intensive exercise can be harmful. For example, jogging can lead to longer-term damage of cartilage of the back and leg joints.

It is much smarter to do MUSCLE BUILDING RESISTANCE EXERCISE on a regular basis. This is particularly useful as we get older. It allows us to focus on our specific body weaknesses.

For example, if your stomach and back muscles need strengthening, lie on your back, bend your knees, and do sit-ups. Start with 20, and add a few more each time, until you reach over 100 per day.

If your legs feel weak, do slow knee bends, or step-ups, or walk stairs every day.

As you get older, focus on your posture; this will help you to both feel and look younger.

Recommended   RESISTANCE   exercise exposure –

- Frequency:	At least every 2nd day
- Intensity:	60% of your maximum
- Time:	30 minutes

8. Choose Your Personal Diet Plan

We can estimate how much overall energy we need in our daily life by starting with the 'BASIC METABOLIC RATE' (BMR). This is the energy we require just to maintain our body, to keep our blood pumping through the veins, to keep breathing, to digest food, and to maintain our body temperature. It varies with body weight, age and gender. Expressed in the old measurement of Calories it adds up as follows:

Typical (BMR) energy use per day: 1,400 cal
Plus walking around the house and to the car: 200 cal
A lazy person's total energy burned: 1,600 cal

It can be as little as that. - On the other hand, if a person eats a breakfast of 500 calories, a burger lunch of 1,000 calories, a dinner with desert and drinks of 2,000 calories, plus a few snacks during the day of 500 calories, this person ends up with a total intake of 4,000 calories a day.

But, if this same person needs only 1,600 calories a day, where do the excess calories go?

We can look at this question again in detail by reviewing the three main nutrients in our food, and their purpose:

- **Proteins** (*e.g., meat, fish, cheese*) - build and maintain our body cells

- **Carbohydrates** (*e.g., sugar, bread, potatos*) - create energy and body reserves
- **Fats** (*e.g., butter, oil, bacon*) - create reserves for future energy production
- Certain other important ingredients have no calories: e.g., **water, fibres, minerals**, etc.

Excess calories in the form of *protein* get eliminated by the body. Our bodies simply cannot store proteins. But, energy producing *carbohydrates* are too vital to get wasted. Why? Our body is still built for the age-old experience of 'feast and famine'. Our body stores reserves for times of food scarcity. How? By converting certain carbohydrates into fat and by building fat pockets, it creates energy storage for future use. But nowadays, the famine part of the equation has dropped off the table.

We need to match our food intake to our energy requirements. This is how we can choose our regime:

1) If we spend most of our days seated or in other ways of low power consumption, we should choose a diet based on **Table 1** above, to avoid gaining weight. Occasionally, you may go to items in Table 2.

If you are currently too heavy and want to shed weight, eat only items from Table 1. It provides a wide and healthy selection.

2) A physically active person can get **sustained energy** from food and drinks in **Table 2** above. For extreme physical exertion, food in **Table 3** may be supplemented for short-term energy.

3) **Table 4** lists food that produces short **energy spikes,** which are **followed by hunger pangs**.
This is extreme junk food that should always be avoided (unless you want to overcome anorexia).

9. S P I R I T

Happiness experts tell us that a key to feeling good is to appreciate what we currently have in life. They tell us to live in the present, to concentrate on our immediate environment and on our experiences as they happen.

This advice applies well to eating and drinking. For each meal, we should select a conducive environment, admire the food presentation, and savour consciously every morsel and every drop we put into our mouth.

Eating is a central activity of human social interaction, from family meals to intimate dates to great feasts and celebrations. Calorie counting and general abstinence inhibit and diminish such positive experiences. It is much wiser to eat selectively, based on the Glycemic Index (GI), thereby enjoying a wide variety and ample quantity of food and drink, without missing out on the fun and without gaining weight.

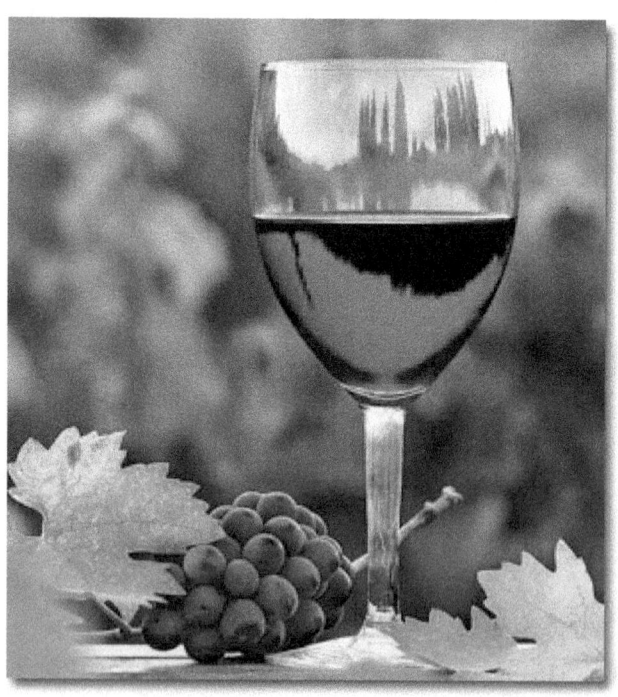

10. CONCLUSION

For less than a hundred years now, we have lived in a very different world from that of our ancestors, with PCs, TVs, cars and airplanes, making up an important part of our advanced society. Our lifestyle has changed drastically, requiring radically less energy output and much lower daily calorie requirements. At the same time, due to changes in food processing technology, our food intake has become much more refined, providing us with a great deal of extra short-term energy and substantially less fibre. These factors combine to give us too much unused body energy, which gets converted and stored as body fat. This is the curse of modern society. Overweight bodies and obesity not only make us feel unhappy and cause severe joint problems, but they can also lead to killer diseases, in particular diabetes 2, heart disease, and cancer.

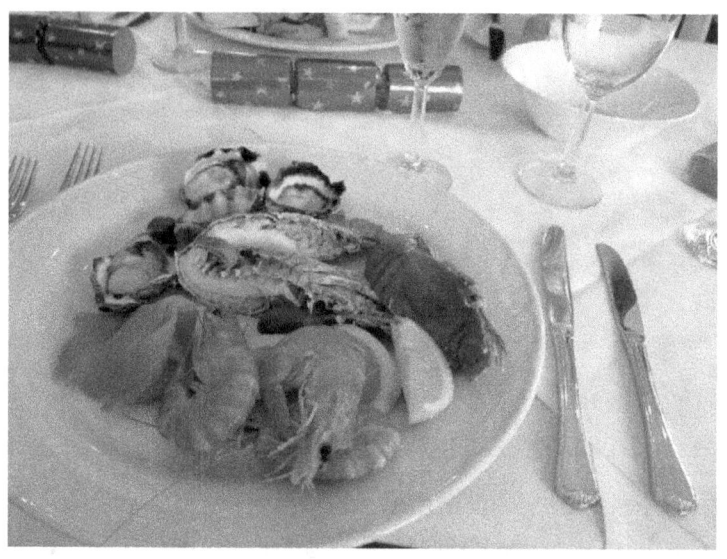

Eating is and should be part of the fun of life! It is the centre of many social activities.

But, eating less is very difficult, because our body makes us want to eat. So, always eating less is not practical. The solution is to eat and drink those foods that do not make us fat. This is possible with the breakthrough of the Glycemic Index (GI). We can eat from all food groups, including carbohydrates, but just not everything.

The GI is a measure that tells us which foods and drinks make us put on weight and which don't.

As a connoisseur, you will find that most of the things you shouldn't eat are the bulk fillers —

in fact, the cheap stuff. You can actually increase your gastronomic delight by following the GI.

Pursuing the advice provided here will bring your weight down and keep it down. It will increase your quality of life.

An ongoing low GI regime, together with a reasonable exercise program, is natural, scientific, and healthy.

Regular 'resistance exercise' and 'detox' round it off.

You will stay in control of your body, keeping it slim, strong and agile. You will feel good about yourself. You will live longer and better.

A low-GI lifestyle liberates you to enjoy the best, here and now! Healthy and enjoyable living is more than a diet. It is a lifestyle.

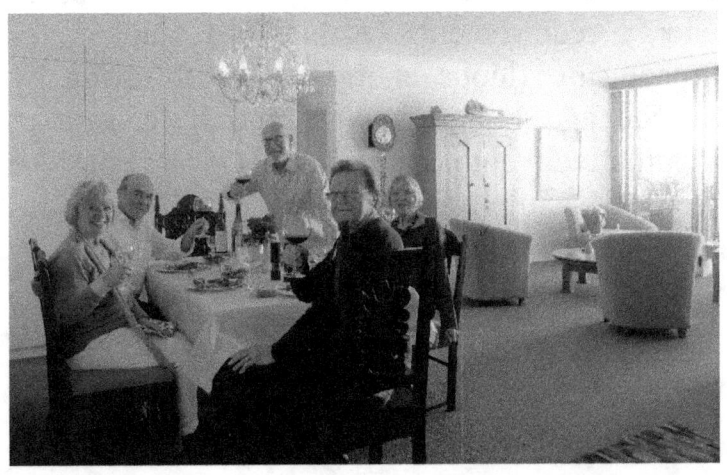

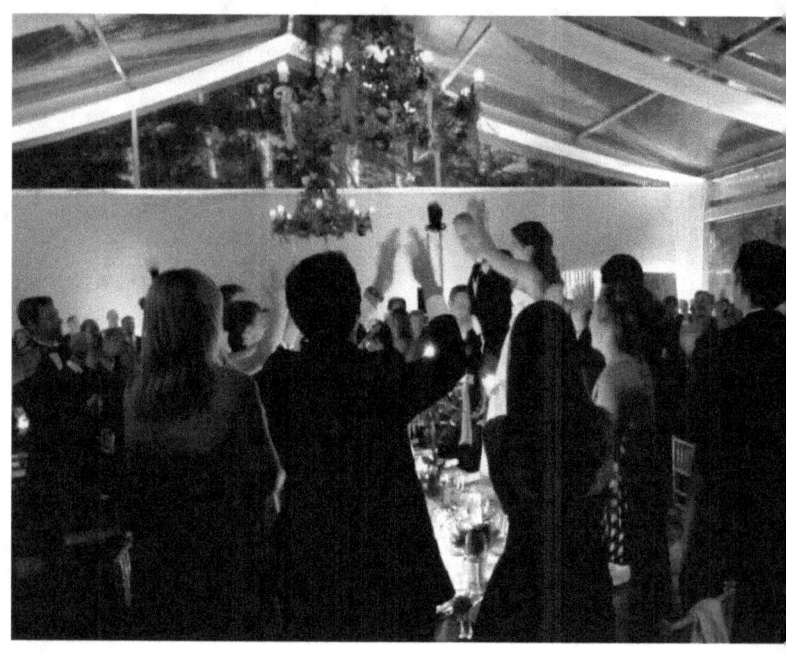

If your weight is appropriate, physically active people need sustained energy.

Choose your diet from the GI range shown in the tables above according to your personal energy requirements. A high GI value gives you a superfluous energy spike, followed by fatigue and hunger pangs, and it leads to a cumulative weight gain. A low GI lets you lose weight, while a medium level provides sustained sports energy.